Barbara Kundig

Yoga Nidra

Blissful deep relaxation

How to approach the challenges of your life in
a relaxed way

Download all audios free of charge with the book

www.blissful-relaxation.com

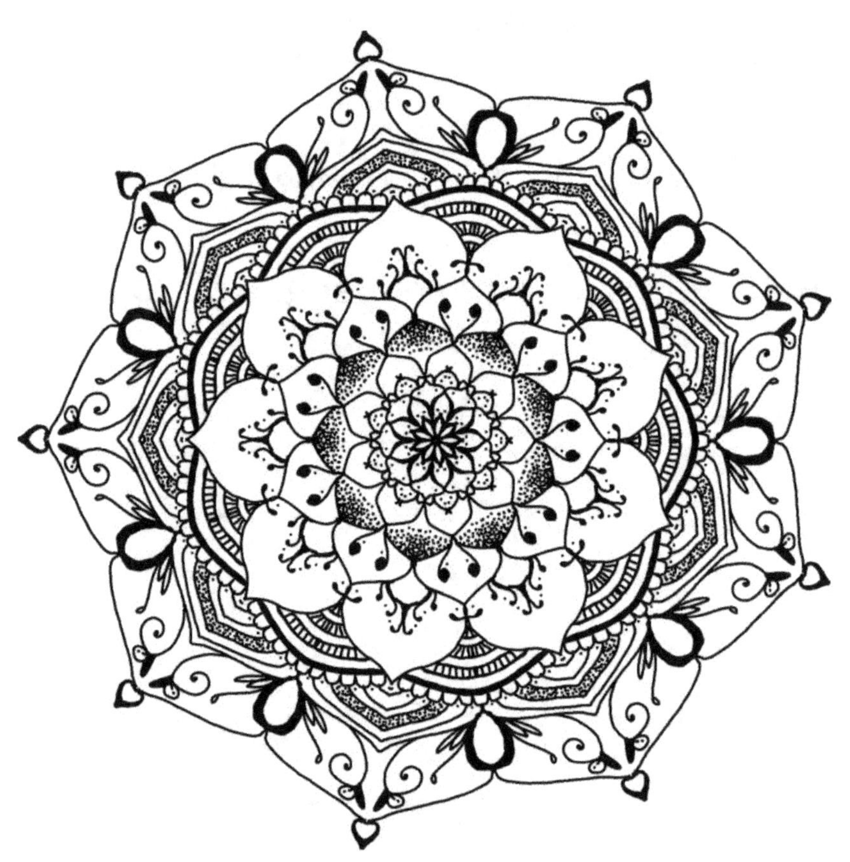

IMPRINT

Yoga Nidra
Blissful deep relaxation
How to approach the challenges of your life in a relaxed way
Barbara Kundig

Author: Barbara Kundig
backoffice@barbara-kuendig.ch

ISBN 978-3-9661079-0-7

About the author

Barbara is a yoga teacher and author of the German bestselling books "Yoga Nidra" (Windpferd Publisher, 2010), "Chakra Yoga Nidra" (Windpferd Publisher, 2014) and "Yoga Nidra for Children" (Windpferd Publisher, 2015) as well as various audios and other books on yoga, relaxation and intuition.

Many of her books have been translated into other European languages.

Furthermore, she is a work and organizational psychologist and holds a Master's degree in business administration.

Barbara has been practicing Yoga Nidra herself for many years on a daily basis.

She has conducted hundreds of classes, workshops and teacher training courses on Yoga Nidra around the world and is very happy to share all her knowledge and experience with you.

She is currently also offering online courses and teacher training courses about Yoga Nidra, intuition and the art of creating an enlightened business..

She is the founder of the Life Mastery Academy and her signature online business program Magic Expansion.

Barbara is a mother of two and a godmother of five wonderful children.

She is a nature lover and can be found in the mountains and on the ski slopes in Switzerland many days of the year.

Learn more about Barbara and her courses at:

www.yoga-nidra.ch

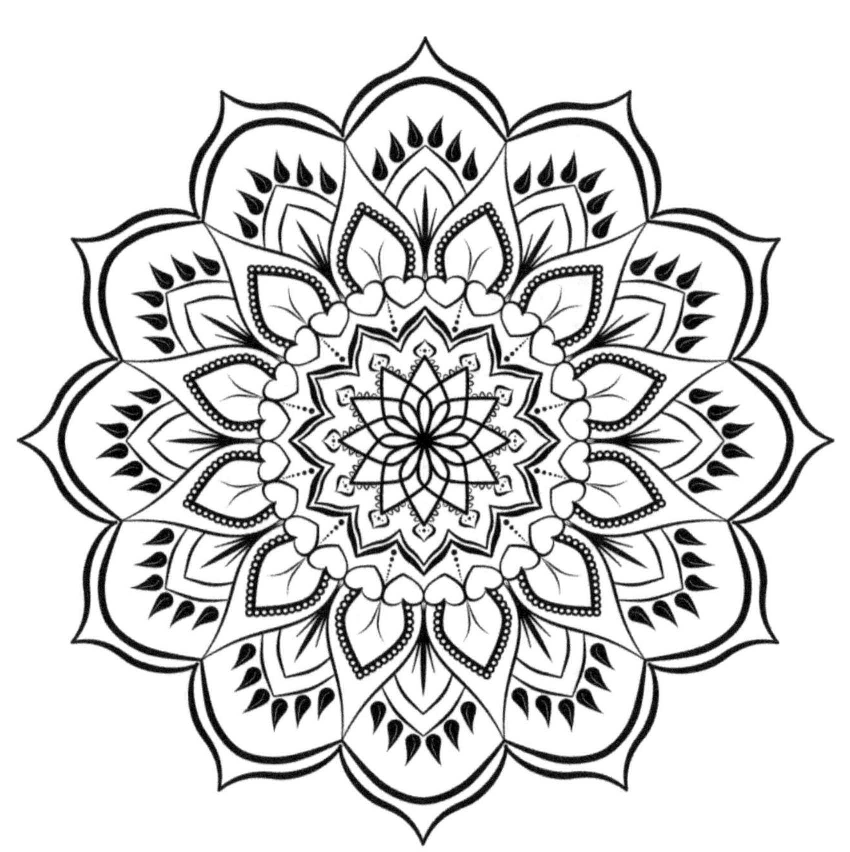

Contents

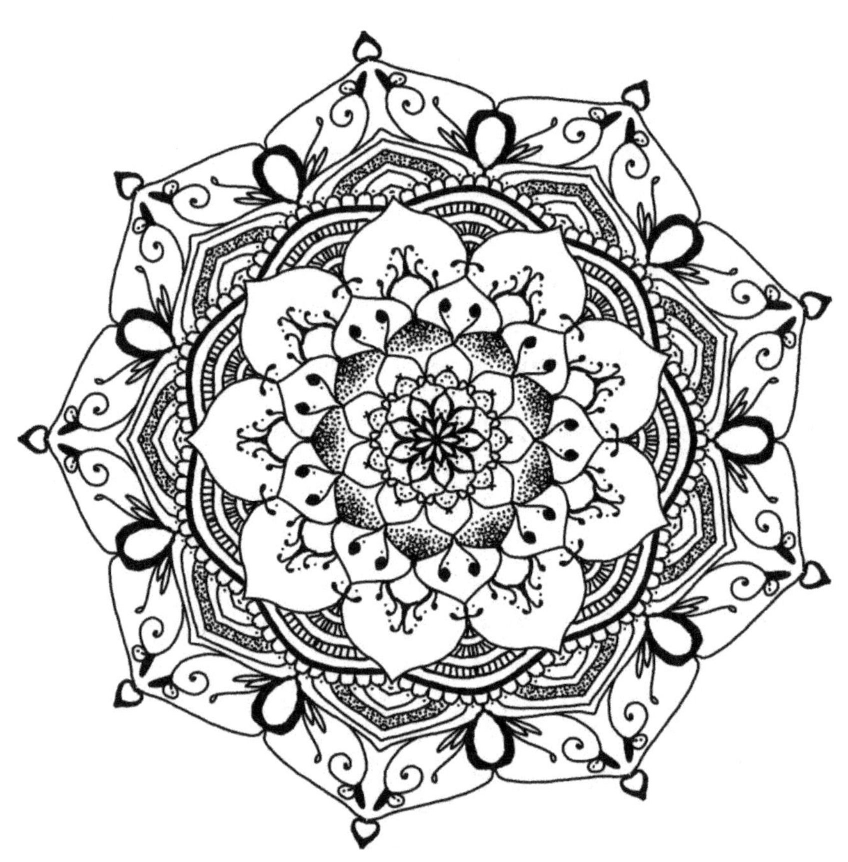

Preface

I was driving to the airport with a light backpack full of light clothing, feeling a bit light-headed. I was finally heading for my yoga teacher training in the country where my mother was born and my grandparents had lived for over 30 years. Finally, I would leave for India. I knew many stories about India, had seen many pictures in my grandmother's countless albums and looked at the countless books in my grandfather's extensive library. I dressed up in saris with my sister and closed my eyes in order not to stare into the tiger's eye that was hanging on the wall at my grandparent's house when I had to go to the bathroom at night. It was a friendly animal during the day but could become terrifying at night to a Swiss girl, growing up in the city. I even ate curry on Christmas Eve when other people would eat traditional local dishes. My grandparents never went back to India after they returned to Switzerland and neither did my mother. But India was very much alive in their house.

I myself had traveled the world in my twenties but somehow never made it to India. Now I felt the urge more than ever. Maybe I would have a family soon and give up some of my freedom to travel. I had a now-or-never feeling, as if something precious would be waiting for me, not to be missed.

I never intended to become a yoga teacher but I was interested in deepening my long personal practice. A very dear friend of mine had already completed her yoga teacher training there and seemed happy when she came back, so why not go to the same place. I signed up, quite some months beforehand, well-organized as I am − or at least I thought I was - and booked a flight. As the departure came closer, I got back to the ashram asking whether they already wanted some money from me. They declined; there was no request for money, since I wasn't on their list... I explained that I was the person who signed up a long time ago and was probably the first on the list... but I wasn't on it and there was no more space for me. Little did I know then... and got a bit upset. What next? Since I had the flight and the weather in Europe did not suggest that a cancellation was an attractive option, I looked for a different ashram that would run a course during the same dates. So there I was on a rainy October morning driving to the airport. Once there, the lady at the check-in counter asked to see my visa. "I don't have one", I replied and looked at my passport with amazement. "Well but you need one...". I was even more amazed. "I cannot let you board the plane". So there I was with my light backpack, wondering what this was all about. Twenty-four hours later, after a run to the travel agency and the embassy and a few funny looks from my family, I finally boarded the plane to Mumbai. Little did I know then that it was all about the blissful relaxation called Yoga Nidra.

One day later, I opened my eyes after my first experience of Yoga Nidra - 30 minutes of blissful relaxation - and knew that this had just been a life-changing experience, something had changed, my focus, my intention, my way of looking at life... I felt bliss.

Quite some years later after having become a mother to two wonderful children, having gathered extensive knowledge and experience of Yoga Nidra, teaching it around the world to thousands of people and having authored a few books, I still feel bliss every day when practicing Yoga Nidra and not only then; it has extended into my daily life.

I am very happy to introduce you to Yoga Nidra and bring bliss into your life.

Namasté!

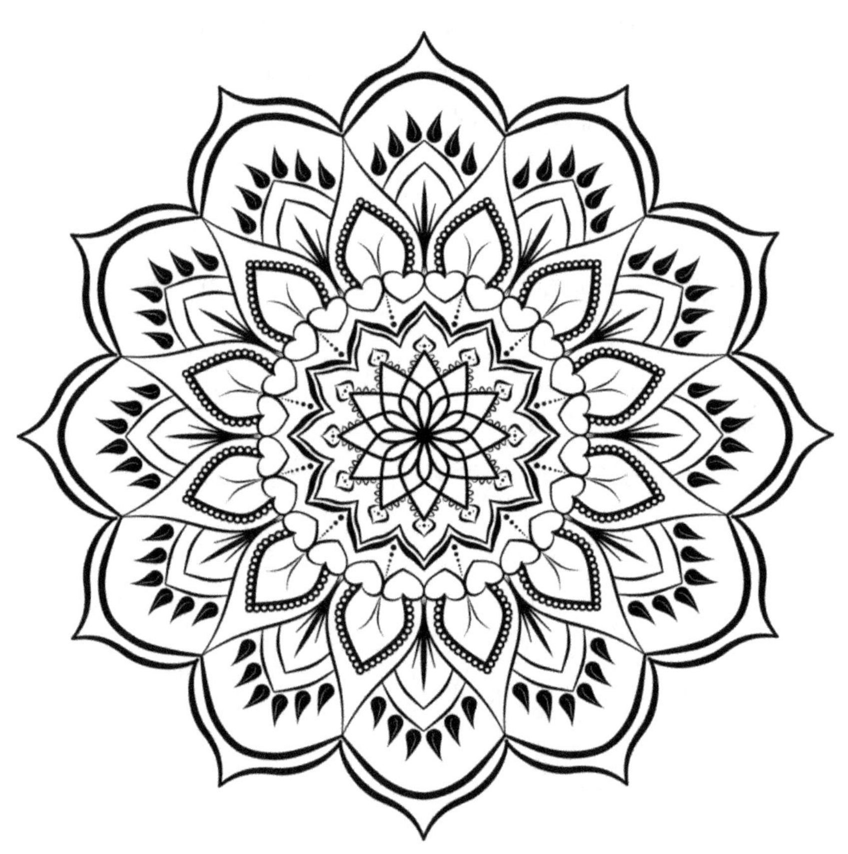

1 - An Invitation to relax!

I invite you to start relaxing right away – there is nothing like a little break from the daily hustle and bustle. All the audios are on a separate website and you are welcome to download them free of charge.

Just go to: www.blissful-relaxation.com

If you are interested in relaxing in a seated position, start with track 1: Perfect chair relaxation.

If you feel like lying down for a shorter but nevertheless valuable relaxation, start with track 2: Serene mat relaxation.

You find the complete version of Yoga Nidra on track 3.

If falling asleep at night is your challenge, start with track 4 - peaceful slumber relaxation -when you are ready to go to bed.

There is nothing you can do wrong, so you can completely give in to the blissful relaxation.

Read and enjoy the information in the book whenever you have time and feel like it. In this way, you will get all the important background information you need to deepen your practice over time and to get the most out of it.

Track 1: Perfect chair relaxation (7 minutes)

If you do not have the possibility to lie down, you can still relax effectively. Practice this exercise in a comfortable sitting position. It is a very effective exercise to practice in the bus or train or in your office chair. Just sit comfortably, close your eyes and follow the instructions. I recommend downloading the track on your phone so that you have got it with you wherever you go.

Track 2: Serene mat relaxation (14 minutes)

You might want to get used to relaxing on a regular basis with a short relaxation practice that you can fit in anywhere and anytime. All you need for the 14-minute practice is a place to lie down – in your home, your office or a hotel room if you are traveling. Anytime during the day is suitable for body and mind to unwind. Make sure you lie down comfortably: on a yoga mat, your bed or a rug. Take a light blanket to cover yourself if you get cold easily. Close the door – you might want to put up a 'Please do not disturb' sign. Play track 2 – your relaxation practice can start.

Track 3: Yoga Nidra (30 minutes)

This is the complete 30-minute Yoga Nidra deep relaxation and meditation practice. Practice it lying on your back, anytime during the day. Since you move between relaxation and half-sleep during Yoga Nidra, this practice has a refreshing and energizing effect. Therefore, do not play this audio too late at night, since the energy you gain from it might disturb your sleep.

Track 4: Peaceful slumber Relaxation (12 minutes)

Put this track on when you are ready to go to sleep. Turn off the light and slip into bed in your pajamas. Listen to the audio and let yourself drift away.

If you are not asleep when the practice is over continue counting backwards from 54. Do not be concerned about not getting enough sleep; if you are still tired in the morning, the 30 minutes of Yoga Nidra will help you to get the necessary energy for your day.

I have also added a bonus text for a Yoga Nidra for healing and self-love in the appendix.

If you are a yoga teacher or a therapist you can use this script for sessions with your clients.

Enjoy!

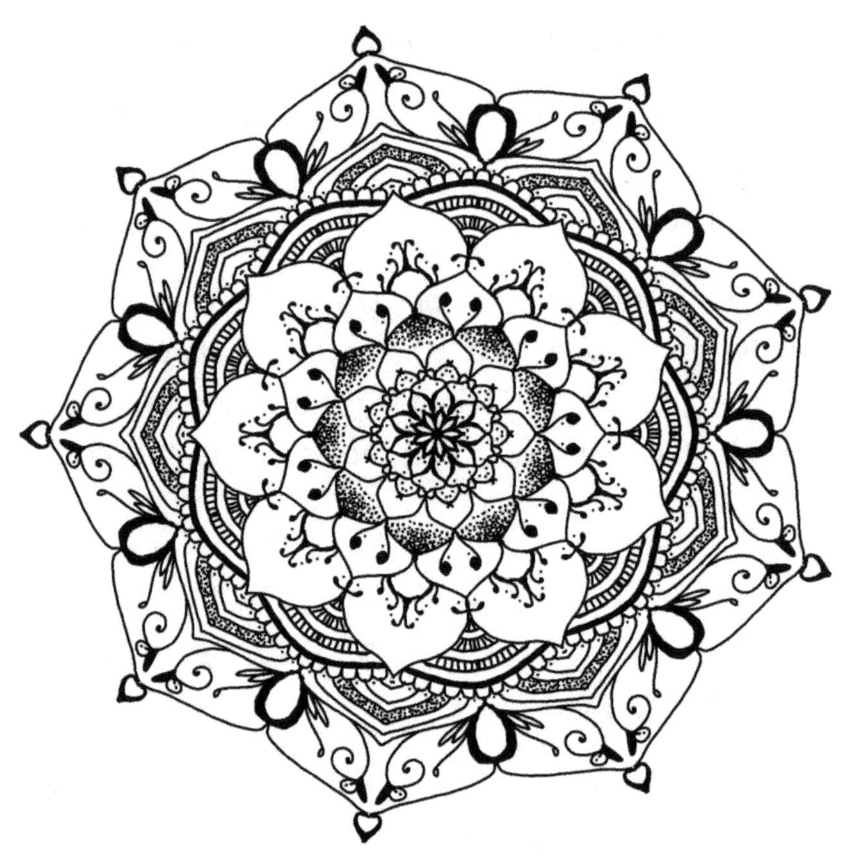

2 - Blissful living

Yoga Nidra is truly a blissful practice!

What positive effects can you expect if you start practicing Yoga Nidra on a regular basis?

Your life seems effortless

Do you ever wish that the things you desire from the bottom of your heart come into your life with ease? That obstacles would dissolve in front of your eyes?

Yoga Nidra gives you the trust and equanimity necessary to jump into the flow of your life. It helps you to understand and see more clearly the things you truly desire and to achieve them with effortlessness.

People who practice Yoga Nidra report that circumstances come into their lives that almost seem miraculous.

Your relationships become more meaningful

Would it help your relationship if you would be more calm, flexible, open to other views?

Yoga Nidra is a tool to develop true calmness that permeates your whole being. If you relax deeply on a regular basis, the waves of your mind will automatically become calm. As a result, you have new possibilities to react to difficult situations.

Yoga Nidra practitioners report that they are sometimes surprised themselves about the positive feedback from people in their surroundings once they have experienced their way of communicating and interacting.

Your health increases

Are you interested in strengthening your immune system, fighting certain illnesses and increasing your general wellbeing?

With the help of Yoga Nidra, you relax not only your body but also your mind and soul. This brings the bodily systems (e.g. the endocrine, cardiovascular, digestive, or nervous system) back into balance as well as all energetic systems (chakras and nadis).

Practitioners are affected significantly less by flu, headaches or insomnia.

Your creativity unfolds

Are you sometimes longing for more inspiration and creativity in various fields of your life? Yoga Nidra will bring that certain spark to it. If you practice Yoga Nidra regularly, you will experience your very own creative way of expressing yourself. You might not become a famous painter straight away but you just have those creative ideas that make your day colorful, playful and spontaneous.

You feel more connected

Are you a spiritual being? Are you looking for meaning and depth in your life?

Yoga Nidra is not only a deep relaxation practice but also a meditation technique. In the depth of the relaxation, you will discover you true Self and feel the connectedness to your surroundings. Your family, colleagues, nature and of course divinity, will become an integral deeply connected part of your life.

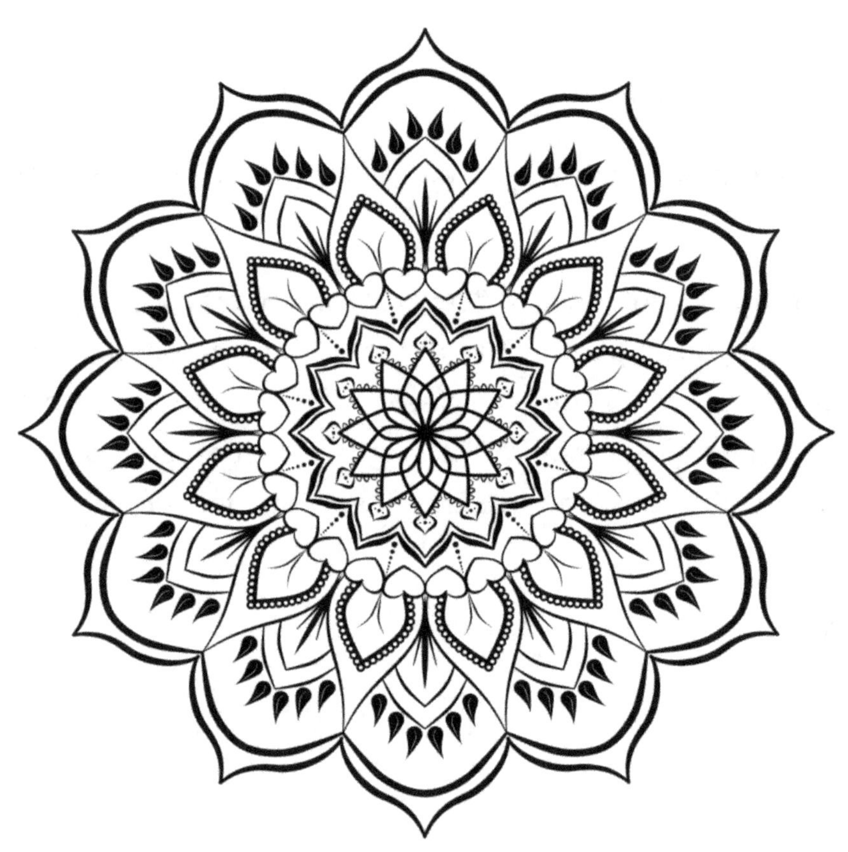

3- Blissful relaxation for blissful living

If we look at our life closely, we realize that most of the time we are in a doing-mode. We rarely approach life in a being-mode. Maybe as an exception: people try to get into the being-mode when they go on holidays or if they get the opportunity to go on extensive travels, while some might even try it on Sundays – or another day off - now and again.

The doing-mode includes a lot of physical activity: our days, weeks, months and years are full of them. We are involved in activities at work, at home with our family and friends. All of them include physical activity. Most of them are one-sided, repetitive and strain the body in one way or another. Much of the time, these physical activities lead to physical tension: we get tense in the shoulders, the neck, or the legs. These tensions can lead to more serious symptoms: headaches, backaches and many more.

How do we break this vicious circle? Often, we do not have the time or do not give it priority to relax our body. In many instances, we only start to do so when the situation already weighs on us quite a bit.

In a blissful life, we relieve ourselves of physical tensions before they can harm us. We relax our body on a daily basis. We do not start by changing our lives fundamentally or by being completely inactive but if we allow our bodies to be in a completely relaxed state once a day, our wellbeing increases significantly.

Once we start relaxing consciously on a regular basis, our body will remember its own blissful state and rediscover its natural tendency to get back to it.

That is blissful living on a physical level.

Eliza:

I love my job as a school teacher and have never found it to be physically strenuous. Nevertheless, a few months ago I developed quite severe neck pain. I did not know whether it was an older story – my doing gymnastics in my teens – or whether it was from sleeping on my side on a mattress which was not exactly new.

Once I started practicing Yoga Nidra on a regular basis, I realized it could have been both. My body was just longing for relaxation and the pain ceased quite quickly.

The doing-mode also has a strong impact on our mind. If there is continuous activity in your life, our mind has to keep up with it. It has to assist the doing-mode and takes on the responsibility by starting to plan the future meticulously. The planning often includes worrying: what if this happens, what if it does not? And it includes trying to make sense of the past by thinking about past events in a detailed manner. The mind moves back and forth between future and past. We worry about what is going to happen with our current job or relationship and we think about what happened to us in our last job or in a relationship for example. As a result, we miss the present moment; it passes without us being aware of it.

In a blissful life, we can quiet the mind when we wish to do so. Our mind is clear and focused and we live in the present moment.

This is blissful living on a mental level.

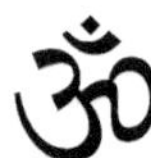

In the doing-mode, we also function in a certain way on the emotional level. We perceive our emotions in a different way than when we are in the being-mode.

In our rushed everyday lives, we tend to get caught up in emotions quicker than we sometimes would like to and we might show tendencies to overestimate their strength. For example, we get really angry because somebody makes an accidental remark about something and we do not realize that hours later the anger still accompanies us.

In a blissful life, we live in harmony with our own emotions. We realize that emotions are like clouds in the sky, in that they come and go as the days pass. We can be with them without getting lost in them.

This is blissful living on an emotional level.

Sophia:

Since I had a car accident 5 years ago, I realized that I was much more worried than before. I saw dangers everywhere. When members of my family went on a trip, I was even dreaming that something would happen to them even though nothing ever happened.

Since I practice Yoga Nidra, I have had many moments without worries and realized that over the last years I worried way too much and lost a lot of energy that way... not any more now!

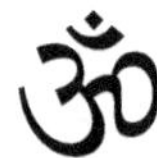

4 – Blissful deep relaxation with Yoga Nidra

That is where Yoga Nidra enters the scene, a deep relaxation and meditation technique for body, mind and soul that leads to profound letting-go and regeneration on all levels: physically, mentally and emotionally.

When practicing Yoga Nidra, a voice will guide you through the different steps of the practice.

A classic Yoga Nidra session always follows a clear structure:

      Preparation
1. Initial relaxation
2. Resolution/Sankalpa
3. Rotation of consciousness
4. Counting backwards
5. Awareness of sensations/Opposites
6. Image visualization
7. Resolution/Sankalpa
8. Closing

Since the relaxation will be very deep and your mind will get in a very relaxed state, you will need an announcement at the end, unless you are a very advanced practitioner.

It is very important that you are comfortable in the position where you lie down for Yoga Nidra, since you will be in this position for 30 minutes without any movements of the body.

This pose is called Shavasana – corpse pose. Please observe the following important details when lying down in Shavasana:

- Turn off your mobile phone completely.
- Take a light blanket, maybe a pillow for under the knees if you have lower back problems.
- Take off your glasses.
- Wear comfortable clothes, take off large and heavy jewellery
- Place your feet a bit more than hip width apart, relax your toes.
- Place your arms away from your body, so that if there was a bit of wind, it could reach the armpits. Turn the palms upwards, relax the fingers.
- Make sure your chin is not too close towards the chest as this restricts the flow of air through your throat. You will be breathing through your nose during the practice of Yoga Nidra.
- Only put a pillow underneath your head if you have neck issues, otherwise the body should lie completely flat on the floor.
- Close your eyes, at the end of the practice you will be asked to open them again.

If you observe those details closely, your body can relax in the best possible way.

If you cannot lie on your back (because of back problems, pregnancy or other reasons) you can lie on the mat in a relaxed pose lying on your side:

Lie on whichever side is more comfortable for you. Straighten the bottom leg. Put the upper foot on the lower knee. Stretch out the lower arm in front of you, palm faces up. Put the upper arm on the side of the body. You can put a pillow under the knee and the head if you would like to. Close your eyes.

Enjoy!

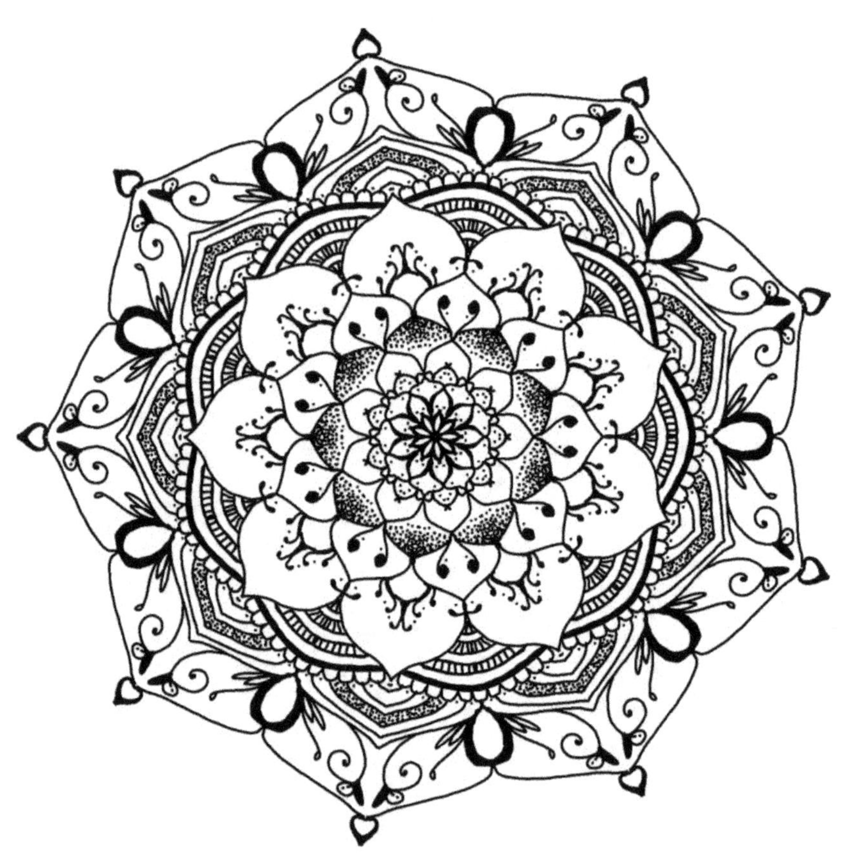

5 – Short relaxation practice

Even though a regular Yoga Nidra sesssion will last half an hour, you can practice shorter relaxation practices to enhance the state of Yoga Nidra – blissful relaxation - in body, mind and soul. The short relaxation practices are perfect little breaks for you.

Perfect Chair Relaxation

This is a 7-minute relaxation practice that can be practiced anytime during the day in a chair, be it at home, in the office or even in the train or plane.

Why?

You might not have a place to roll out your mat. Or you want to get into the habit and be able to relax wherever you are.

When?

You can practice the perfect chair relaxation any time during the day, be it as an attunement in the morning, as a break in the train or in the office chair after lunch or on the sofa rather than watching TV.

What to consider?

Try to relax the body as best as you can. Of course, you still have to use some muscles to sit more or less straight but you can relax your legs, arms and hands, shoulder and neck as well as the whole face.

What to expect?

Expect to react more calmly during the following activities. You will make your decision with a clearer mind and you will be more focused.

Serene Mat Relaxation

This is a 14-minute practice that can be practiced anytime during the day if you have an opportunity to lie down, be it in bed or on a mat or a carpet.

Why?

This is a good break if you are keen to relax your body, maybe because you are tired, feel a bit sick or have pain somewhere in your body. It is also valuable to start feeling more comfortable in your body in general. It is also a wonderful opportunity to learn how to let go of any tension in the body that might arise because of your physical activities.

When?

Practice the serene mat relaxation any time during the day if you have a mat at your disposal.

What to consider?

Be aware that there is no need for a nicely decorated yoga room. You can put your mat on the floor anywhere. Ensure that the floor is not too cold, otherwise it might be a good idea to place a blanket under the mat and to have another one ready to cover your body.

What to expect?

This practice will give you a lovely sense of relaxation and a calm state of mind in a short time. You will come out of the practice in a focused and calm way.

What to expect?

You will start to appreciate the comfortable relaxed feeling in your body and mind, and you will realize that the effects will last throughout the rest of the day.

Peaceful Slumber Relaxation

This is a 12-minute practice especially designed for the nighttime.

Why?

Since the full practice of Yoga Nidra might give you too much energy if practiced in the evening, this is the prefect practice if you have difficulties falling asleep at night or do not sleep well.

When?

Practice right before you go to sleep in your pajamas ready to sleep. Turn the lights off already.

What to consider?

Position yourself in your bed in a way that you do not need to get up again after the practice. Make sure that there is plenty of fresh air in the room or leave the window open for the night. You might want to arrange some relaxing music after the audio.

What to expect?

This practice will help you drift into sleep. You might dream more intensely.

Look forward to feeling more energetic and equanimous in the morning.

27

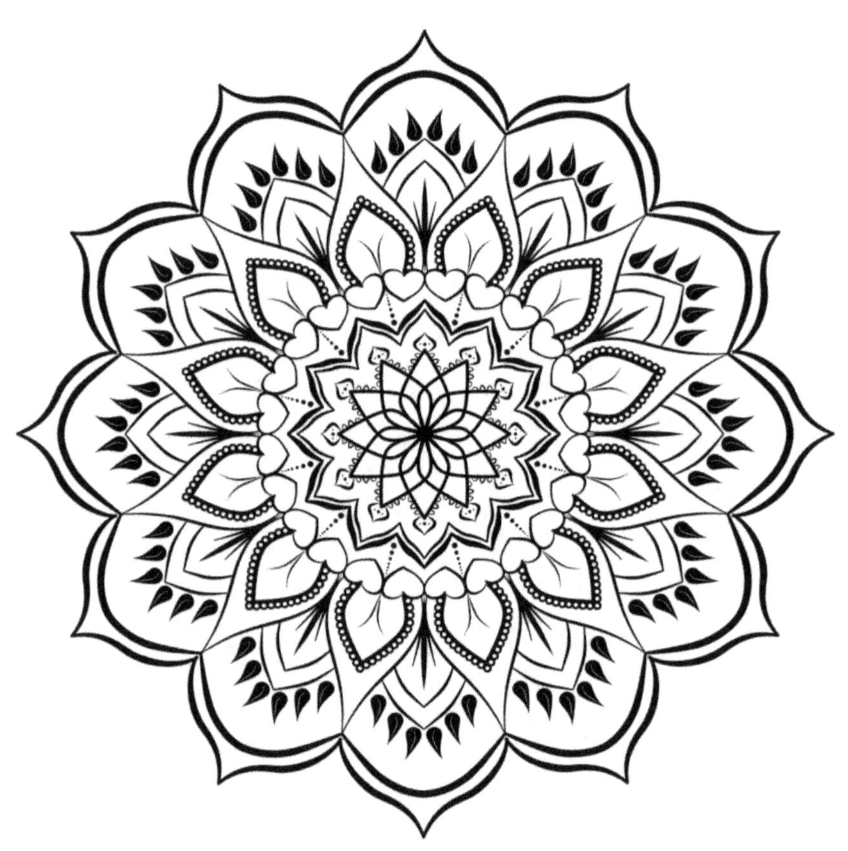

6 - Yoga Nidra – step by step

In this chapter, you will learn about all the different techniques that you find in a Yoga Nidra session. This gives you the necessary knowledge to deepen your experiences during the practice. You will see that over time your personal practice will change and deepen and that you will grow on all levels of your existence.

Preparation

> Practice Yoga Nidra lying on your back, on a yoga mat, your bed or on a rug in the yogic relaxation pose called Shavasana. In this pose, the body should be straight from head to toe, the legs slightly apart and the arms a little away from the body, the palms of the hands are turned upwards.

> If you cannot lie on your back (because of back problems, pregnancy or other reasons), lie down in the relaxed pose lying on one side.

> It is important not to move during the practice, otherwise the relaxation will diminish. If you move your arm to scratch your forehead for example, the muscles in the arm will contract and will take a while to relax completely again. There is no reason to worry, however, if you get so distracted during the practice that you have to get up (e.g. when your baby is crying or you are waiting for a truly urgent call).

Cover yourself if you tend to get cold quickly. You can put a pillow under your knees or a rolled towel if you have lower back issues. In severe cases, you could even put your feet and calves on a chair. Only put a pillow under the head if you have head or neck issues.

Yoga Nidra is always practiced with closed eyes. At the end of the practice, you will be asked to open your eyes again.

My additional recommendation:

> *Be aware of how you lie down when going to sleep at night. Do this as consciously as when you practice Yoga Nidra. Give your body the perfect opportunity to relax completely for the following hours. Lie down comfortably so you do not have to move later on because you put too much strain on certain parts of your body, for example the shoulders, the neck or the hips. Lying on your back is a good position for going to sleep since it puts the least strain on your body.*

1. Initial relaxation
    It is very normal for the mind to become agitated once you lie down. It is as if the mind says: now there is space so I can make myself heard... You can (and should) practice Yoga Nidra even if you do not feel calm, your mind will calm down through the practice. Do not get caught in a thought or a story though; just let those thoughts pass by like clouds in the sky. Be gentle with them but firm. You can do this by mentally saying to the thoughts: I know you would like to get attention, but I am practicing Yoga Nidra right now, so you'll have to wait please...
    This attitude and training of the mind will make the mind quieter during the rest of the day.

Whenever you get the opportunity during your day: pause for a moment and check what your thoughts are doing. Just notice, do not judge or wish it would be different. Observe how thoughts arise and pass by.
Then just bring your attention back to your breath in order to quiet the mind. Observe how your abdomen rises when you breathe in and falls when you breathe out.

2. Resolve/Sankalpa

In every Yoga Nidra sequence, you are asked to make a resolve, also called Sankalpa. Your Sankalpa should be in accordance with your innermost immaterial desires. You might want to take some time away from your Yoga Nidra practice and listen to your heart or your soul to see what it is that you long for. You might want to write it down so you are clear about your Sankalpa. Once you know your Sankalpa, use it for at least three weeks. Then see what has changed in your life and whether the Sankalpa is still the right one. It can take a few weeks or months until you feel that it is time to change it. It is not a matter of time but a matter of your feeling comfortable with your Sankalpa and the way your life unfolds.

It is important that your Sankalpa is always short, positive and in the present.

Examples could be:

"I live my life in peace" or

"I am calm" or

"Body and mind are in perfect harmony".

My additional recommendation:

> *Repeat your Sankalpa internally whenever you think of it – while brushing your teeth, cooking, waiting for the train...*
>
> *You might want to write it down nicely on a piece of paper and put it in your purse or wallet or stick it to the fridge.*

3. Rotation of consciousness

   When you relax your limbs, the respective motor areas in your brain relax at the same time since there is a direct connection with the physical limbs and their place on the motor cortex in the brain.

   It is important that your awareness rotates quite quickly in order to get the energy (prana in yogic terms) flowing through your body. When starting with the practice, it might be difficult to really feel the single limbs. This will improve with practice.

> *Remember that wherever your attention goes into your body, relaxation will follow and energy will flow there. Use this principle if you want to relieve yourself from pain in the neck or back, PMS, or any other ailment.*
> *Just move your attention to the place where relaxation is desired… and be aware of the soothing effect that your awareness causes.*

4. Breathing and counting

    You are asked to observe your breath while counting backwards from 27. Counting backwards helps the body and mind relax more and more - as opposed to counting upwards. The number 27 is a quarter of 108 which is a number with great significance in yogic traditions. The meditation mala (garland) has 108 beads, there are said to be 108 marma points (vital points) in ayurvedic medicine, and there are 108 upanishads (certain yogic scriptures). It is also a number that symbolizes wholeness: the Sun, the Moon and the Earth are connected by this number, the average distance from the Sun and the Moon to the earth is 108 times their diameter.

    The numbers 54 and 27 (108 divided by 2 and then again divided by 2) are said to have the same powerful effects.

    While counting backward from 27 four times, you observe the breath at the navel, chest, and nostrils in turn. By doing so, you offer the mind a point of concentration. At the same time, you help the energy moving through the body in an upward direction, from the lower to the higher chakras.

It is important to count in the rhythm of your natural breath. At different times, you will count back to different numbers. If you breathe quickly you will get to 1, whereas if you breathe in a more relaxed manner you might count until 17 for example.

5. Image visualization

   In Yoga Nidra, great emphasis is put on cleaning and balancing the chakras, therefore allowing spiritual energy to flow through the body freely. Chakras are subtle energy centers along the spine that can be felt at the front and back of the body and also in the subtle energy field of the body. The functioning of your chakras represents how you deal with fundamental themes of your existence.

   You are asked to visualize a series of images – which represent the symbols of the chakras - in quite a quick manner. Try to develop a vision of them on all levels: feelings, awareness, and imagination.

The following table gives you an overview of the chakras:

Symbol in Yoga Nidra	Chakra	Bija mantra	English name	Location in the body	Theme
Fireplace with a burning fire	Sahasrara	-	Crown chakra	On the top of the head	Higher consciousness, spirituality
Bright eye	Ajna	Om	Third eye	Between the eyes	Intuition, higher knowledge
Cold drops of nectar	Visuddhi	Ham	Throat chakra	Throat	Communication, expression
Tiny flame of light on a small lamp	Anahata	Yam	Heart chakra	Center of the chest	Love, compassion
Bright yellow sunflower	Manipura	Ram	Solarplexus	Upper abdomen	Energy, will
Waves on a vast ocean at night	Svadhisthana	Vam	Sexual chakra	Lower abdomen	Sexuality, creativity
Inverted red triangle	Mooladhara	Lam	Base chakra	Base of the spine	Life force, trust

While you visualize the symbols in Yoga Nidra, your energy centers are cleaned and balanced. This will have a positive effect on your overall wellbeing and personal development.

My additional recommendation:

> *If a certain chakra is not as balanced as you would like it to be, repeat its Bija mantra silently for yourself, or even say it out aloud.*
>
> *You can also do this before an important event. For example, if you prepare yourself for a presentation, repeat 'Ham' to strengthen your communication skills, or if you are not clear about a decision you have to take, repeat 'Om' in order to strengthen your intuition.*

6. Awareness of sensations/Opposites

   In this part, you are asked to feel contrary sensations in your body (heaviness-lightness, cold-heat, pain-pleasure). This helps harmonize the opposite brain hemispheres, with the right hemisphere representing the more emotional and intuitive processes and the left one representing the more rational processes. This technique also relieves memories of profound feelings. For example, if you still have the memory of a physical or emotional pain stored somewhere in your body – consciously or unconsciously – it will be released. Ultimately, feeling the opposites regularly and in quite a quick manner, will help you overcome duality. In daily life, we are often caught within the opposites, if it is warm we would like it be cold and vice versa, if we feel pain we want it to be over, if we feel pleasure we are scared that it will pass. This technique will help you become more accepting of situations and life in general, without resisting it or wanting to change it.

My additional recommendation:

Get the flexibility to distance yourself from strong emotions if they become overwhelming. You can work with a scale from 10 to 1. Determine how strong the emotion is for you: 10 is the strongest, 1 is the weakest value. Then try to lessen the emotion by distancing yourself from it a bit. Just try to get one number lower, then 2 until you feel more comfortable with the emotion. In this way, you become more and more emotionally flexible.

7. Resolve/Sankalpa
   The Sankalpa is always repeated at the end of Yoga Nidra to reinforce its effects.

8. Closing
   Please start moving you body slowly and take time getting up. The muscles have been completely relaxed, blood pressure and pulse have dropped during the practice. It is therefore important to give your circulation the chance to restart slowly.
   In this way, you can benefit most from the fresh energy that started flowing through your body and mind during Yoga Nidra.

My additional recommendation:

> *Get into the habit of stretching regularly – like cats do. Stretch yourself thoughtfully and with pleasure when you get up in the morning; start your internal engine. Also do it as a short break during the day. Take a few moments to refuel.*

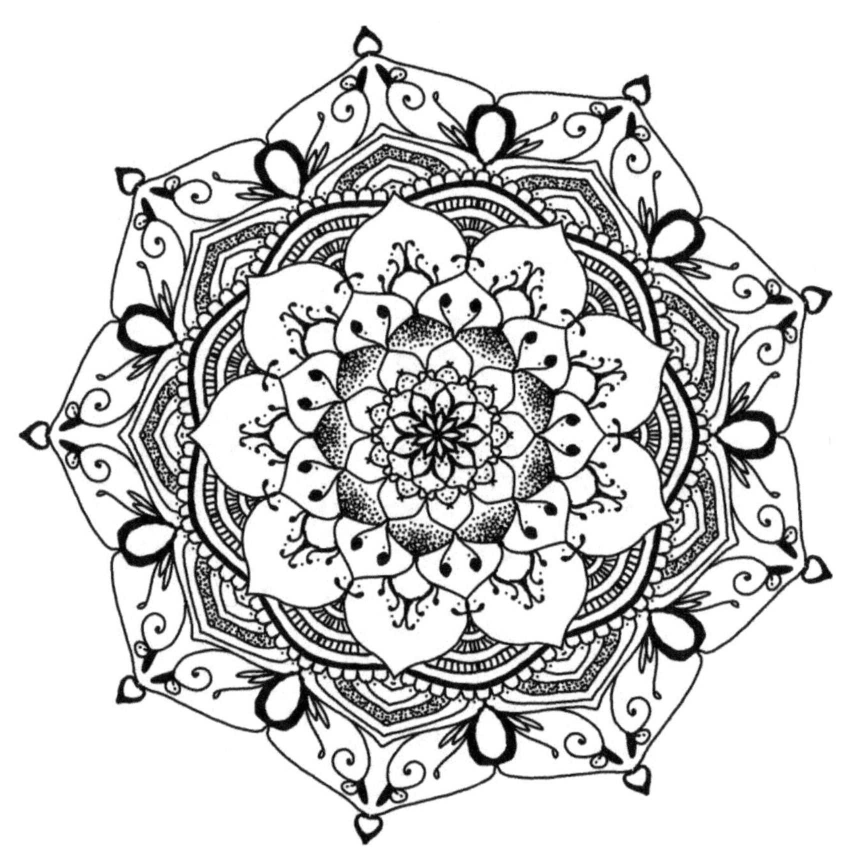

7 - Yoga Nidra and the brain

What happens in your brain while you relax?

Obviously, when you relax there will be less activity in your brain so your brainwave pattern slows down. Technically speaking, it moves from Beta to Alpha state, or even Theta state in Yoga Nidra.

We can differentiate between four different major brainwaves patterns which can be measured with en EEG (electroencephalogram):

Name	Frequency	Stage of wake or sleep	Experiences
Beta	13-30 cycles per second	Waking state	Awake, mind is active
Alpha	8-12 c.p.s.	Relaxation	Relaxed, mind is active but quiet
Theta	4-7 c.p.s.	Half-sleep, slumber, border between waking state and sleep	Sleepy, mind is still receptive though not proactive
Delta	0-4 c.p.s.	Deep sleep	Sleeping, mind is not active

When practicing a regular relaxation technique, the brainwave pattern will move from the "regular" waking state – Beta - to Alpha.

When practicing Yoga Nidra, you move from Beta to Alpha first. This is relaxation. With the practice unfolding during the half hour, you start to go even deeper and move between Alpha and Theta, the relaxed state and a state of slumber where you are extremely relaxed with the mind still being receptive.

Yoga Nidra becomes a tightrope walk with shares of Alpha and Theta. The amount of Alpha and Theta will be different every time you practice Yoga Nidra, which is one reason why you will have a different experience every time.

If you have the impression that you fell asleep during Yoga Nidra, your brainwaves showed the Theta pattern. That is the reason why your body and mind regenerate very much, as if one had slept for a few hours. Remember that it is not deep sleep though. In deep sleep your brain shows Delta waves, even slower than Theta.

The practice is set up that way that you do not come into the Delta phase. Throughout the practice, you will be reminded to stay awake, meaning not to go into a Delta brainwave pattern. In the end, when you are asked to move hands and feet and to open the eyes again, it is a gentle coming back to Beta state; you are awake and fresh.

Emily:

When I started to practice Yoga Nidra, I sometimes had the impression that I missed half of the practice. Nevertheless, I got so much more equanimous at work that I realized that even though I did not hear the Sankalpa consciously, it must have a very strong concrete effect.

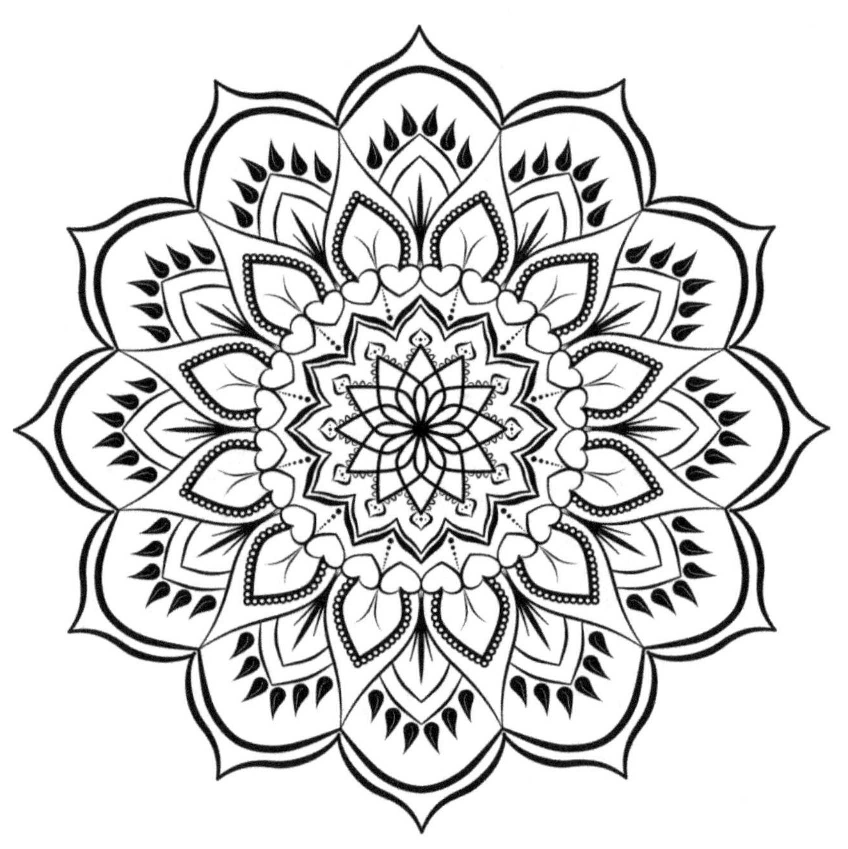

8 – Yoga Nidra – the subconscious and the supraconscious

It might happen to you that images appear in your mind anytime during the practice of Yoga Nidra. This can be gentle and subtle images or impressions or they can seem more prominent or pushy to you. Allow any images to appear.

On the one hand, those images can be released from your subconscious mind. If you see such images, it feels as if you know parts of them already, have seen them before or know the feelings associated with those images. You might feel uncomfortable about them since they remind you of unpleasant memories. If such images appear, you can free yourself from the negative imprints they might have on you by just letting them surface and then dissolve.

On the other hand, images might appear from the supraconscious mind. Those images can feel like flashes of intuition and can be very clear and strong. In addition, they can also be new or surprising and can have quite an impact on the course of your life, since they bring you valuable information about questions you might have or about the next steps to take.

Just be attentive but do not dwell on the images during your Yoga Nidra practice. You can think about the meaning of those images after the practice or you can meditate on them later on.

Carlos:

I kept getting images of my grandparents' house during Yoga Nidra. I realized that my feelings about those images were ambiguous – sometimes it made me happy and sometimes sad. It then dawned on me that both were true: I was and still am happy about having had such a warm and loving childhood but on the other hand, there is a sadness in me that those times are definitely over.

Lisa:

As an art director of a magazine, I was very curious from the beginning to learn how to get images from my supraconscious mind during Yoga Nidra. It took some time since I really had to learn how to relax physically and mentally first. But with time, I learnt how to perceive the subtle but clear and enormously helpful images that give me insight about the topics I should cover in my magazine.

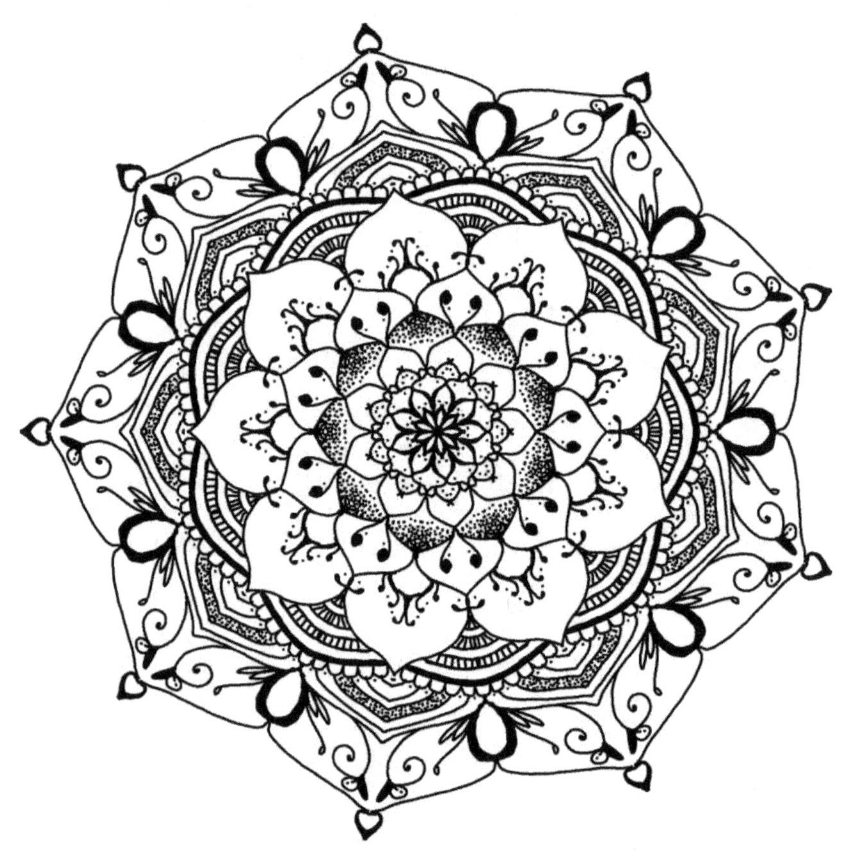

9 – My wish for you

I hope you enjoyed this book and the audios.

I hope you like the idea of blissful living.

And I do hope that living blissfully will become your reality.

This is what I wish for you from the bottom of my heart.

Love and light,

Barbara

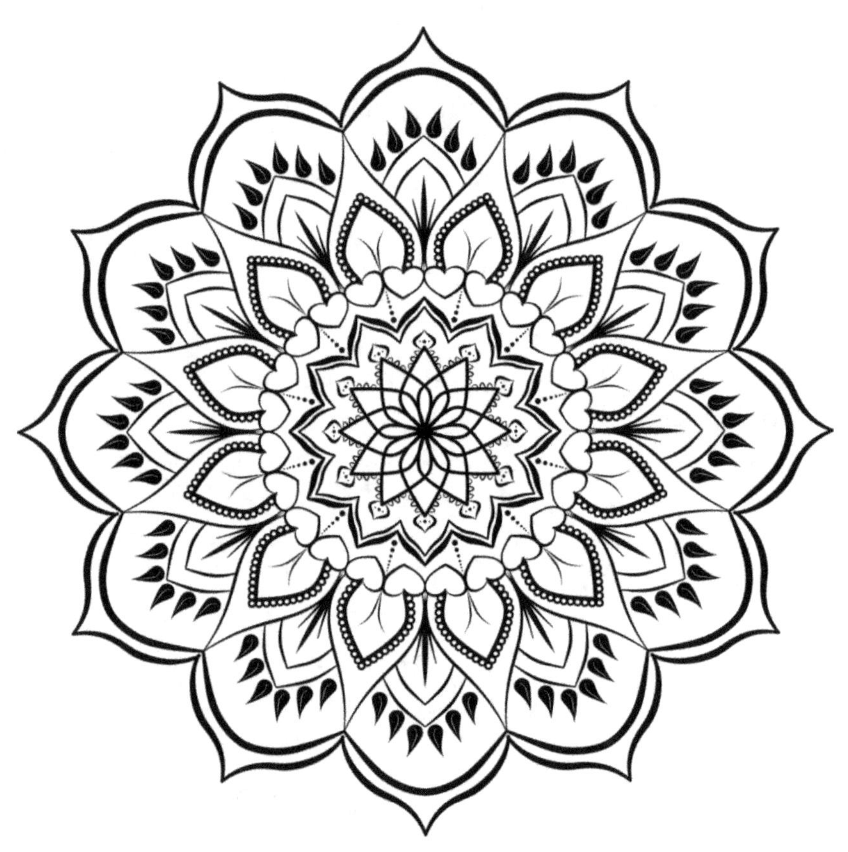

Appendix

Perfect chair relaxation

(Length: 7 minutes)

Welcome to a short relaxation practice in a sitting position that will refresh you on a physical, mental and emotional level.

Please sit down comfortably.

Close your eyes and keep them closed until you are told to open them.

Take a deep breath and as you breathe out feel all your worries flow out of you.

Now bring your attention to the following parts of your body: Your feet, legs, abdomen, chest, back, hands, arms, shoulders, neck, head.

Your body is completely relaxed.

Now bring your attention to the natural breath, become aware that you are breathing quietly and slowly.

Now become aware of the breath through the nostrils, the natural breath flowing through both nostrils and meeting in the eyebrow center to form a triangle.

Feel the breath flowing through both nostril and uniting in the eyebrow center.

Now start to practice mental awareness of breathing through alternate nostrils counting backwards from 27, as follows: 27 inhale through the left nostril, 27 exhale through the right nostril, 26 inhale through the right nostril, 26 exhale through the left nostril, 25 inhale through the left nostril, 25 exhale through the right nostril and so on.

Continue the practice and repeat the numbers mentally.

Now develop awareness of your physical existence.

Become aware of your arms and legs and your whole body.

Now develop awareness of the room, walls, ceiling, noises in the room and noises outside.

Take your mind out, become completely external.

Sit quietly for a few moments and keep your eyes closed.

Start moving your body and stretching yourself, please take your time, do not hurry.

When you are sure that you are wide awake, open your eyes.

Enjoy your fresh and relaxed state.

Serene mat relaxation

(Length: 14 minutes)

Welcome to a short relaxation practice that will refresh you on a physical, mental and emotional level.

Please lie down on your back.

The body should be straight from head to toe, the legs slightly apart and the arms a little away from the body, the palms of the hands are turned upwards.

Adjust everything, your body, position and clothes, until you are completely comfortable.

Close your eyes and keep them closed until you are told to open them.

Take a deep breath and as you breathe out feel all your worries flow out of you.

Now become aware of sounds in the distance, become aware of the most distant sounds that you can hear.

Search out distant sounds and follow them for a few moments.

Move your attention from sound to sound.

Gradually bring your attention to closer sounds, to sounds outside this building, and then to sounds inside this building.

Now develop your awareness of this room.

Without opening your eyes visualize the four walls, the ceiling, your body lying on the mat, see your body lying on the mat.

Become aware of the existence of your physical body lying in stillness, total awareness of your body lying in total stillness.

Now begin rotation of consciousness, rotation of awareness by taking a trip through the different parts of the body.

As quickly as possible your awareness is to go from part to part.

Keep yourself alert but do not concentrate too intensely.

Become aware of the right hand, right hand thumb, second finger, third finger, fourth finger, fifth finger, palm of the hand, back of the hand, the wrist, the lower arm, the elbow, the upper arm, the shoulder, the armpit, the right waist, the right hip, the right thigh, the kneecap, the calf muscle, the ankle, the heel, the sole of the right foot, the top of the foot, the big toe, second toe, third toe, fourth toe, fifth toe.

Now become aware of the left hand, left hand thumb, second finger, third finger, fourth finger, fifth finger, palm of the hand, back of the hand, the wrist, the lower arm, the elbow, the upper arm, the shoulder, the armpit, the left waist, the left hip, the left thigh, the kneecap, the calf muscle, the ankle, the heel, the sole of the left foot, the top of the foot, the big toe, second toe, third toe, fourth toe, fifth toe.

Now go to the back. Become aware of the right shoulder blade, the left shoulder blade, the right buttock, the left buttock, the spine, the whole back together.

Now go to the top of the head, the forehead, both sides of the head, the right eyebrow, the left eyebrow, the space between the eyebrows, the right eyelid, the left eyelid, the right eye, the left eye, the right ear, the left ear, the right cheek, the left cheek, the nose, the tip of the nose, the upper lip, the lower lip, the chin, the throat, the right chest, the left chest, the middle of the chest, the navel, the abdomen.

The whole of the right leg, the whole of the left leg, both legs together. The whole of the right arm, the whole of the left arm, both arms together. The whole of the back, buttocks, spine, shoulder blades, the whole of the front, abdomen, chest, the whole of the back and front together, the whole of the head, the whole body together, the whole body together, the whole body together.

Now concentrate your awareness on the movement of your navel area, concentrate on your navel movements. Your navel is rising and falling slightly with every breath, with each and every breath it expands and contracts. Concentrate on this movement in synchronization with your breath.

Go on practicing and be sure that you are aware.

Now start counting your breaths backwards from 27, like this: 27 navel rising, 27 navel falling, 26 navel rising, 26 navel falling, 25 navel rising, 25 navel falling, and so on. Repeat the numbers mentally to yourself as you continue counting your breaths.

Now develop awareness of your physical existence.

Become aware of your arms and legs and your body lying on the mat.

Now develop awareness of the room, walls, ceiling, noises in the room and noises outside.

Take your mind out, become completely external.

Lie quietly for a few moments and keep your eyes closed.

Start moving your body and stretching yourself, please take your time, do not hurry.

When you are sure that you are wide awake, open your eyes and sit up slowly.

Enjoy your fresh and relaxed state.

Yoga Nidra

(Length: 30 minutes)

Welcome to the practice of Yoga Nidra.

Please lie down on your back.

The body should be straight from head to toe, the legs slightly apart and the arms a little away from the body, the palms of the hands are turned upwards.

Adjust everything, your body, position and clothes, until you are completely comfortable.

During Yoga Nidra, there should be no physical movement.

Close your eyes and keep them closed until you are told to open them.

Take a deep breath and as you breathe out feel the worries of the day flow out of you.

Try to stay awake during Yoga Nidra. Make a resolution to yourself now: 'I will remain awake throughout the practice.'

During Yoga Nidra, you are functioning on the levels of hearing and awareness, and the only important thing is to follow the voice. Do not analyze the instructions as this will disturb your mental relaxation. Simply follow the voice with total attention and feeling, and if thoughts come to disturb you from time to time, let them go and continue the practice. Allow yourself to become calm and steady.

Now bring about a feeling of inner relaxation in the whole body. Concentrate on the body and become aware of the importance of complete stillness. Develop your awareness of the body from the top of the head to the tips of the toes. Complete stillness and complete awareness of the whole body. Continue your awareness of the whole body, the whole body, the whole body...

At this moment, you should make your resolve. The resolve has to be very simple. Try to discover one naturally. It should be a short, positive statement in simple language.

Repeat your resolve three times with awareness, feeling and emphasis.

The resolve you make during Yoga Nidra is bound to come true in your life.

Now begin rotation of consciousness, rotation of awareness by taking a trip through the different parts of the body. Your awareness is to go from part to part as quickly as possible. Repeat the part in your mind and simultaneously become aware of that part of the body. Keep yourself alert but do not concentrate too intensely.

Become aware of the right hand, right hand thumb, second finger, third finger, fourth finger, fifth finger, palm of the hand, back of the hand, the wrist, the lower arm, the elbow, the upper arm, the shoulder, the armpit, the right waist, the right hip, the right thigh, the kneecap, the calf muscle, the ankle, the heel, the sole of the right foot, the top of the foot, the big toe, second toe, third toe, fourth toe, fifth toe.

Become aware of the left hand, left hand thumb, second finger, third finger, fourth finger, fifth finger, palm of the hand, back of the hand, the wrist, the lower arm, the elbow, the upper arm, the shoulder, the armpit, the left waist, the left hip, the left thigh, the kneecap, the calf muscle, the ankle, the heel, the sole of the left foot, the top of the foot, the big toe, second toe, third toe, fourth toe, fifth toe.

Now go to the back. Become aware of the right shoulder blade, the left shoulder blade...the right buttock, the left buttock...the spine...the whole back together...

Now go to the top of the head. The top of the head, the forehead, both sides of the head, the right eyebrow, the left eyebrow, the space between the eyebrows, the right eyelid, the left eyelid, the right eye, the left eye, the right ear, the left ear, the right cheek, the left cheek, the nose, the tip of the nose, the upper lip, the lower lip, the chin, the throat, the right chest, the left chest, the middle of the chest, the navel, the abdomen...

The whole of the right leg, the whole of the left leg, both legs together. The whole of the right arm, the whole of the left arm, both arms together. The whole of the back, buttocks, spine, shoulder blades, the whole of the front, abdomen, chest, the whole of the back and front together, the whole of the head, the whole body together, the whole body together, the whole body together.

Please do not sleep. Total awareness, no sleeping, no movement. The whole body on the floor, become aware of your body lying on the floor. Your body is lying on the floor, see your body lying perfectly still on the floor, in this room. Visualize this image in your mind.

Become aware of your breath. Feel the flow of your breath in and out of your lungs. Do not try to change the rhythm, the breathing is natural, automatic, you are not doing it, there is no effort. Maintain awareness of your breath. Continue: complete awareness of breath.

Now concentrate your awareness on the movement of your navel area, concentrate on your navel movements. Your navel is rising and falling slightly with every breath, with each and every breath it expands and contracts. Concentrate on this movement in synchronization with your breath. Go on practicing, but be sure that you are aware.

Now start counting your breaths backwards from 27, like this: 27 navel rising, 27 navel falling, 26 navel rising, 26 navel falling, 25 navel rising, 25 navel falling, and so on. Say the numbers mentally to yourself as you count your breaths. If you make a mistake, go back to 27 and start again.

Now stop your counting of the navel breath and shift your attention to the chest, please shift to the chest. Your chest is rising and falling slightly with each and every breath, become aware of this. Continue concentrating on the movement of the chest and start counting backwards from 27, in the same way as before: 27 chest rising, 27 chest falling, 26 chest rising, 26 chest falling, 25 chest rising, 25 chest falling, and so on. Again repeat the words and the numbers mentally to yourself as you count. No mistakes, if you make a mistake go back to the start again, to 27. Keep on with the practice, counting and awareness, awareness and counting.

Stop counting and go to the nostrils, become aware of the breath moving in and out of the nostrils. Concentrate on the movement of the breath in and out of the nostrils and start counting as before, you know it very well by now, 27 breathing in, 27 breathing out. Complete awareness please, continue counting, no mistakes.

Keep on with the practice, continue.

Stop your counting and leave your breathing and start visualization. The symbols of the chakras, the subtle energy centers of your body, will be named. Try to develop a vision of them on all levels... feelings, awareness, emotion, imagination, as best you can.

The symbol for mooladhara chakra at the perineum is a red inverted triangle, a red inverted triangle...

The symbol for swadhistana chakra at the base of the spine is waves on a vast ocean at night, waves on a vast ocean at night...

The symbol for manipura chakra behind the navel is a bright yellow sunflower, a bright yellow sunflower...

The symbol for anahata chakra behind the heart is a tiny flame of light on a small lamp, a tiny flame of light on a small lamp...

The symbol for vishuddi chakra at the throat is cold drops of nectar, cold drops of nectar...

The symbol for ajna chakra at the top of the vertebral column is a bright eye, a bright eye...

The symbol for sahasrara chakra at the crown of the head is a fireplace with a burning fire, a fireplace with a burning fire...

Now awaken the feeling of heaviness in your body, the feeling of heaviness. Become aware of heaviness in every single part of the body. You are feeling so heavy that you are sinking into the floor. Awareness of heaviness, awareness of heaviness.

Now awaken the feeling of lightness in your body, awaken the feeling of lightness. A sensation of lightness and weightlessness in all parts of the body. Your body feels so light that it seems to be floating away from the floor. Awareness of lightness, awareness of lightness.

Now recollect an experience of pain, concentrate and try to remember the experience of pain. Any pain you have experienced in your life, mental or physical, recollect the feeling of pain.

Now recollect a feeling of pleasure, any kind of pleasure, physical or mental. Recollect this feeling and relive it, make it vivid... awaken the feeling of pleasure.

Now is the time to repeat your resolve... repeat the same resolve that you made at the beginning of the practice, do not change it...

repeat the resolve three times with full awareness and feeling.

Relax all efforts, draw your mind outside and become aware of your breathing, become aware of the natural breath.

Awareness of the whole body, and awareness of breathing. Your body is lying totally relaxed on the floor...

You are breathing quietly and slowly. Develop awareness of your body from the top of the head to the tips of the toes.

Become aware of the floor, and the position of your body lying on the floor... visualize the room around you, become aware of your surroundings.

Lie quietly for some time and keep your eyes closed.

Start moving your body and stretching yourself.

Please take time, do not hurry.

When you are sure that you are wide awake open your eyes and sit up slowly.

Enjoy your fresh and relaxed state.

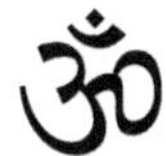

Peaceful slumber relaxation

(Length: 12 minutes)

Welcome to a relaxation practice that can be practiced before going to sleep. Please lie down comfortably in your bed. Turn off the light. Adjust everything, your body, position, pajamas and linen until you are completely comfortable. Close your eyes and keep them closed. Take a deep breath and as you breathe out, feel all your worries flow out of you.

Now become aware of distant sounds. Move your attention from sound to sound, listening only, do not try to analyze. Bring your attention closer, become aware of sounds outside the building; then become aware of sounds inside the building, inside this room. Develop awareness of this room...the walls, the ceiling, your body lying in bed. See your body lying in bed and become aware of your physical existence. Now become aware of your natural breath, total awareness of your natural breath. Feel how you become more and more relaxed.

Now begin rotation of consciousness, rotation of awareness by taking a trip through the different parts of the body:

Become aware of the right hand, right hand thumb, second finger, third finger, fourth finger, fifth finger, palm of the hand, back of the hand, the wrist, the lower arm, the elbow, the upper arm, the shoulder, the armpit, the right waist, the right hip, the right thigh, the kneecap, the calf muscle, the ankle, the heel, the sole of the right foot, the top of the foot, the big toe, second toe, third toe, fourth toe, fifth toe.

Become aware of the left hand, left hand thumb, second finger, third finger, fourth finger, fifth finger, palm of the hand, back of the hand, the wrist, the lower arm, the elbow, the upper arm, the shoulder, the armpit, the left waist, the left hip, the left thigh, the kneecap, the calf muscle, the ankle, the heel, the sole of the left foot, the top of the foot, the big toe, second toe, third toe, fourth toe, fifth toe.

Now go to the back. Become aware of the right shoulder blade, the left shoulder blade, the right buttock, the left buttock, the spine, the whole back together.

Now go to the top of the head. The top of the head, the forehead, both sides of the head, the right eyebrow, the left eyebrow, the space between the eyebrows, the right eyelid, the left eyelid, the right eye, the left eye, the right ear, the left ear, the right cheek, the left cheek, the nose, the tip of the nose, the upper lip, the lower lip, the chin, the throat, the right chest, the left chest, the middle of the chest, the navel, the abdomen.

The whole of the right leg, the whole of the left leg, both legs together. The whole of the right arm, the whole of the left arm, both arms together. The whole of the back, buttocks, spine, shoulder blades, the whole of the front, abdomen, chest, the whole of the back and front together, the whole of the head, the whole body together, the whole body together, the whole body together.

Become aware of the right hand, right hand thumb, second finger, third finger, fourth finger, fifth finger, palm of the hand, back of the hand, the wrist, the lower arm, the elbow, the upper arm, the shoulder, the armpit, the right waist, the right hip, the right thigh, the kneecap, the calf muscle, the ankle, the heel, the sole of the right foot, the top of the foot, the big toe, second toe, third toe, fourth toe, fifth toe.

Become aware of the left hand, left hand thumb, second finger, third finger, fourth finger, fifth finger, palm of the hand, back of the hand, the wrist, the lower arm, the elbow, the upper arm, the shoulder, the armpit, the left waist, the left hip, the left thigh, the kneecap, the calf muscle, the ankle, the heel, the sole of the left foot, the top of the foot, the big toe, second toe, third toe, fourth toe, fifth toe.

Now go to the back. Become aware of the right shoulder blade, the left shoulder blade, the right buttock, the left buttock, the spine, the whole back together.

Now go to the top of the head. The top of the head, the forehead, both sides of the head, the right eyebrow, the left eyebrow, the space between the eyebrows, the right eyelid, the left eyelid, the right eye, the left eye, the right ear, the left ear, the right cheek, the left cheek, the nose, the tip of the nose, the upper lip, the lower lip, the chin, the throat, the right chest, the left chest, the middle of the chest, the navel, the abdomen.

The whole of the right leg, the whole of the left leg, both legs together. The whole of the right arm, the whole of the left arm, both arms together. The whole of the back, buttocks, spine, shoulder blades, the whole of the front, abdomen, chest, the whole of the back and front together, the whole of the head, the whole body together, the whole body together, he whole body together.

Now draw your attention to the natural ingoing and outgoing breath. Feel the breath moving along the passage between the navel and the throat. On inhalation it rises from the navel to the throat, on exhalation it descends from the throat to the navel. Be completely aware of the respiration, navel to throat, throat to navel. Do not try to force the breath, just awareness. Maintain your awareness and at the same time start counting your breaths backwards as follows: 'Breathing in: 54, breathing out: 54, breathing in: 53, breathing out: 53, breathing in: 52, breathing out: 52.' And so on, from 54 to 1. Count to yourself mentally as you follow the rise and fall of your breath from navel to throat and back again. Total awareness of breathing and counting. The breathing is slow and relaxed. Please continue counting, the breathing is slow and relaxed. You are completely relaxed, you are completely relaxed, complete relaxation in body mind and soul, complete relaxation.

Bonus Text

Yoga Nidra for Healing and Self-Love

(Lengths: 30 Minutes)

Welcome to the practice of Yoga Nidra.

Please lie down on your back.

The body should be straight from head to toe, the legs slightly apart and the arms a little away from the body, the palms of the hands are turned upwards.

Adjust everything, your body, position and clothes, until you are completely comfortable.

During Yoga Nidra, there should be no physical movement.

Close your eyes and keep them closed until you are told to open them.

Take a deep breath and as you breathe out feel the worries of the day flow out of you.

Try to stay awake during Yoga Nidra. Make a resolution to yourself now: 'I will remain awake throughout the practice.'

During Yoga Nidra, you are functioning on the levels of hearing and awareness, and the only important thing is to follow the voice. Do not analyze the instructions as this will disturb your mental relaxation. Simply follow the voice with total attention and feeling, and if thoughts come to disturb you from time to time, let them go and continue the practice. Allow yourself to become calm and steady.

Now bring about a feeling of inner relaxation in the whole body. Concentrate on the body and become aware of the importance of complete stillness. Develop your awareness of the body from the top of the head to the tips of the toes. Complete stillness and complete awareness of the whole body. Continue your awareness of the whole body, the whole body, the whole body...

Now repeat the following sentence, your resolve, three times:

I am whole and bathed in self-love.

The resolve you make during Yoga Nidra is bound to come true in your life.

We now begin rotation of consciousness, rotation of awareness by taking a trip through the different parts of the body. As quickly as possible the awareness is to go from part to part. Repeat the part in your mind and simultaneously become aware of that part of the body. Keep yourself alert but do not concentrate too intensely. Become aware of the right hand. (pause)

Right hand thumb, second finger, third finger, fourth finger, fifth finger, palm of the hand, become aware of your palm, back of the hand, the wrist, the lower arm, the elbow, the upper arm, the shoulder, the armpit, the right waist, the right hip, the right thigh, the kneecap, the calf muscle, the ankle, the heel, the sole of the right foot, the top of the foot, the big toe, second toe, third toe, fourth toe, fifth toe...

Become aware of the left hand thumb, second finger, third finger, fourth finger, fifth finger, palm of the hand, become aware of your palm, back of the hand, the wrist, the lower arm, the elbow, the upper arm, the shoulder, the armpit, the left waist, the left hip, the left thigh, the kneecap, the calf muscle, the ankle, the heel, the sole of the left foot, the top of the foot, the big toe, second toe, third toe, fourth toe, fifth toe...

Now to the back. Become aware of the right shoulder blade, the left shoulder blade...the right buttock, the left buttock...the spine...the whole back together...

Now go to the top of the head. The top of the head, the forehead, both sides of the head, the right eyebrow, the left eyebrow, the space between the eyebrows, the right eyelid, the left eyelid, the right eye, the left eye, the right ear, the left ear, the right cheek, the left cheek, the nose, the tip of the nose, the upper lip, the lower lip, the chin, the throat, the right chest, the left chest, the middle of the chest, the navel, the abdomen...

The whole of the right leg...the whole of the left leg...both legs together. (pause) The whole of the right arm... the whole of the left arm...both arms together. (pause) The whole of the back, buttocks, spine, shoulder blades...the whole of the front, abdomen, chest...the whole of the back and front...together...the whole of the head...the whole body together...the whole body together...the whole body together...

Now become aware of the subtle physical meeting points between the body and the floor. Feel the meeting points (longer pause)

Please do not sleep. Total awareness, no sleeping, no movement. The whole body on the floor, become aware of your body lying on the floor. Your body is lying on the floor, see your body lying perfectly still on the floor, in this room. Visualize this image in your mind.

Become aware of your breath. Feel the flow of your breath in and out of your lungs. Do not try to change the rhythm, the breathing is natural, automatic, you are not doing it, there is no effort. Maintain awareness of your breath. Continue: complete awareness of breath.

Now concentrate your awareness on the movement of your navel area, concentrate on your navel movements. Your navel is rising and falling slightly with every breath, with each and every breath it expands and contracts. Concentrate on this movement in synchronization with your breath. Go on practicing but be sure that you are aware.

Now start counting your breaths backwards from 27 while observing the movements of your navel.

Now stop your counting of the navel breath and shift your attention to the chest, please shift to the chest. Your chest is rising and falling slightly with each and every breath, become aware of this. Continue concentrating on the movement of the chest and start counting backwards from 27, in the same way as before.

Stop counting and go to the nostrils, become aware of the breath moving in and out of the nostrils. Concentrate on the movement of the breath in and out of the nostrils and start counting as before. *(2 minutes pause)*

Now awaken the feeling of heaviness in your body, the feeling of heaviness. Become aware of heaviness in every single part of the body. You are feeling so heavy that you are sinking into the floor. Awareness of heaviness, awareness of heaviness.

Now awaken the feeling of lightness in your body, awaken the feeling of lightness. A sensation of lightness and weightlessness in all parts of the body. Your body feels so light that it seems to be floating away from the floor. Awareness of lightness, awareness of lightness.

Now start visualization.

See a beautiful flower in your heart center.

From this flower golden light flows to you.

Feel the energy flowing inside into your body, your mind, your soul.

Feel the warm and beautiful love flowing generously inwards.

Now imagine a stream white light flowing through your whole body from the universe.

A pillar of white light.

The white light is bringing healing into your whole body, your mind and your soul.

Feel the healing energy flowing through your whole being. (long pause, 2-8 minutes)

Now is the time to repeat your resolve three times:

I am whole and bathed in self-love.

Relax all efforts, draw your mind outside and become aware of your breathing, become aware of the natural breath. Awareness of the whole body, and awareness of breathing. Your body is lying totally relaxed on the floor... you are breathing quietly and slowly. Develop awareness of your body from the top of the head to the tips of the toes. Become aware of the floor, and the position of your body lying on the floor... visualize the room around you, become aware of your surroundings.

Lie quietly for some time and keep your eyes closed.

Start moving your body and stretching yourself.

Please take time, do not hurry.

When you are sure that you are wide awake open your eyes and sit up slowly.

Enjoy your fresh and relaxed state.

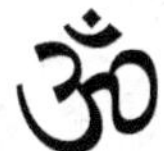

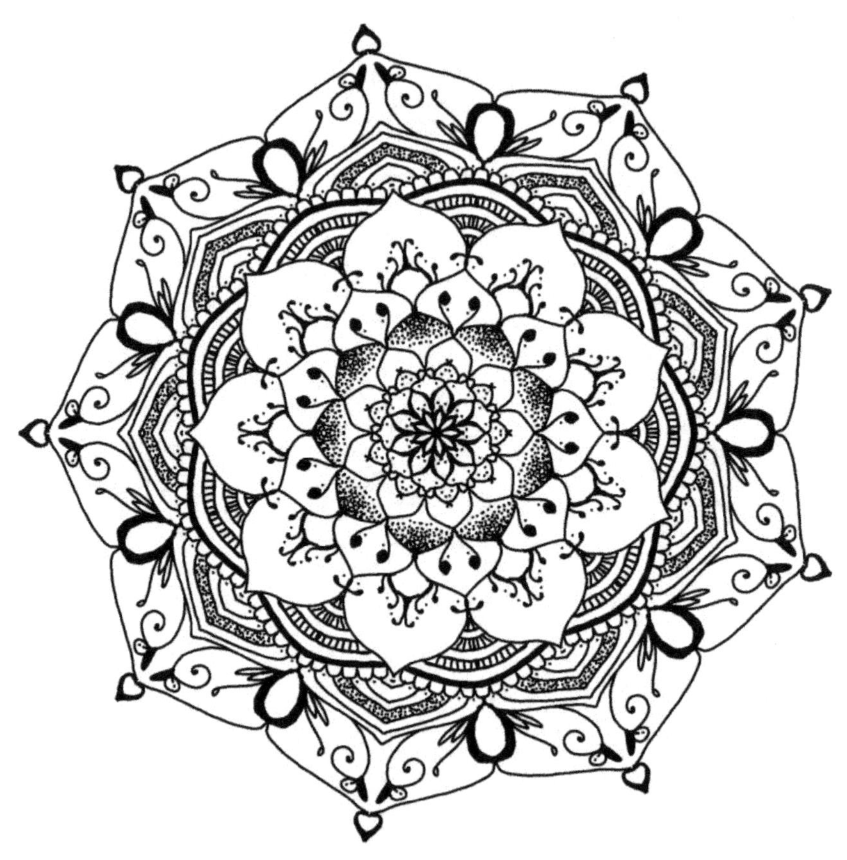

Publications by Barbara

1. Kündig, Barbara: Yoga Nidra; Book and CD/Audio;
   Windpferd Verlag; 2010.

   ISBN 978-3-89385-637-4

2. Kündig, Barbara: Yoga-Inspiration; Card set;
   Windpferd Verlag; 2011.

   ISBN 978-3-89385-665-7

3. Kündig, Barbara: Yoga Nidra; CD/Audio;
   Windpferd Verlag; 2012.

   ISBN 978-3-86410-001-7

4. Kündig, Barbara/Sinclair, Marta: Intuitiv richtig – wir
   wissen mehr als wir denken (Intuition – We Know More
   than We Think); Book and CD/Audio;
   Windpferd Verlag; 2012;

   ISBN 978-3-86410-022-2

5. Kündig, Barbara: Schwangerschafts-Yoga (Prenatal Yoga);
   Book and CD/Audio;
   Trias Verlag; 2013.

   ISBN 978-3-83046-654-3

6. Kündig, Barbara/Hirschi, Gertrud: RückenYoga (Yoga for
    the Back); Book and DVD;
    Trias Verlag; 2014.

    ISBN 978-3-83046-911-7

7. Kündig, Barbara: Chakra Yoga Nidra; Book and CD/Audio;
    Windpferd Verlag; 2014.

    ISBN 978-3-86410-081-9

8. Kündig, Barbara/Schluep, Barbara: Yoga Nidra für Kinder
    (Yoga Nidra for Children); Book and CD/Audio; Windpferd
    Verlag; 2015.
    ISBN 978-3-86410-098-7

9. Kündig, Barbara: Yoga Asanas; Book;
    Windpferd Verlag; 2015.
    ISBN 978-3-86410-108-3

10. Kündig, Barbara: Life Mastery, 12 Schritte zu
    vollkommener Gelassenheit; Book and CD/Audio;
    Windpferd Verlag; 2018.
    ISBN 978-3-86410-187-8

11. Kündig, Barbara: Life Mastery, Das Arbeitsbuch:
    Vollkommene Gelassenheit in 12 Schritten umsetzen;
    Book, Windpferd Verlag; 2019.
    ISBN 978-3-86410-201-1

12. Kündig, Barbara: Das Universum kennt deinen Weg, 12
    universelle Gesetze, die dein Leben auf zauberhafte Weise
    beeinflussen (The Universal Laws); Book; Windpferd
    Verlag; 2020.
    ISBN 978-3-86410-226-4